Embracing the Moment

Embracing the Moment

Living With, Through & Beyond Cancer

Patricia Carley

While the incidents in this book did happen, some of the names and personal characteristics of some of the individuals have been changed. Any resulting resemblance to persons living or dead is entirely coincidental and unintentional.

Author photo by Erin Pihlaja
Cover and book design by Melissa Mykal Batalin

Printed in the United States of America

The Troy Book Makers • Troy, New York • thetroybookmakers.com

To order additional copies of this title,
contact your favorite local bookstore or visit www.tbmbooks.com

ISBN: 978-1-61468-044-4

for Marilyn

Acknowledgements

I wish to acknowledge the following people who helped me through this challenging time.

My family and friends who prayed for me and cared for me during my surgeries, treatments and recovery; the healers and practitioners of alternative therapies who gave me the spiritual energy and emotional strength to carry on; the nurses, doctors, technicians and support staff who used their skills to help my body heal; and my fellow-travelers on the journey of living with, through and beyond cancer.

Thank you for helping me to embrace the moment.

Foreword

Let me start by saying this is not a handbook on "How to Survive Cancer."

It is not about "How To Beat Cancer by Eating Special Foods."

It is not about "Winning the War Against Cancer."

I did not use those phrases while experiencing cancer. I did not let anyone around me use words that depicted violent images nor let them pressure me into trying 'designer' cures.

I ate the foods that gave me comfort and gained 15 pounds during chemotherapy and radiation treatments.

I accepted the experience Spirit had handed me and learned to welcome the lessons it taught me.

In August, 2005 I was diagnosed with two cancers: breast and colon. I was told they were each a primary site which is good news in the cancer business. After countless tests, CAT/PET scans, bone scans, X-Rays, biopsies, surgeries both minor and major, post-cancer treatments, medications that made me vomit, others to stop the vomiting, and blood test after blood test, I am still here to tell the tale.

I had Reiki treatments, massages and facials on a regular basis and shamanic ceremonies, novenas and prayers said to and for me.

I practiced Tai Chi and Yoga in bed when I was too weak, and upright when I felt stronger; visualized perfect health and eventually became well.

I believe it was the blending of these two styles of healing: western allopathic medicine and alternative, complimentary healing practices that manifested a cure in me.

This book is not about "Getting Cancer and Finding God" although this is exactly what happened to me. I was cracked open, shattered and reduced to my elements so Spirit could come in.

Everywhere I looked during my hospital stay and subsequent treatments I saw God at work in my life.

I learned to embrace whatever moment I was in and let God/ Spirit guide my steps to a full recovery.

Diagnosis: Cancer

Cancer: Signified by the Crab in Western Astrology. It is the faintest Zodiacal constellation in our night sky. It holds the Beehive cluster which is recognizable by eyesight as a blurry blob, at best.

Cancer: A water sign. Ruler of the emotions. Fluid, flowing, cascading, seeping its way into all the nooks and crannies of the body. It buzzes like a beehive busily making a honeycomb in the organs, blood and bones.

Cancer: It is a crab scuttling along at the bottom of the sea with feelers and claws, its pincers reaching out and grasping and not letting go. It has a hard shell or soft, a protective covering in either case. Warding off its enemies with a shield.

Cancer: Growing, spreading, reaching out its tentacles in my body, surrounding itself in my left breast with a soft-shell, protective, fatty shield. In my large intestine as a tumor readying itself to burst through the wall into my abdominal cavity.

Cancer: Lurking, growing silently, stealthily for probably years, showing itself here and there as a clot of blood, a lump in my left underarm, a pain in my lower left side. As fatigue and a sharp pain in my abdomen on a sunny afternoon when I have yard work to do but go back to bed instead.

Cancer: The diagnosis that strikes fear in every patient's heart when they hear the word directed towards them.

It is August 9, 2005 and I am about to begin a month of rude awakenings and miracles. A time for looking deep within myself to find the strength to live through another night and greet the dawn with hope.

I have been overcome with a migraine for three days that no medication can touch. I am weak from not eating, dehydrated, the pain in my left side is worse and I can feel lumps both there and in my left breast. I have a friend drop me off at the hospital on her way to work and my journey begins.

In the ER I wait and wait to be seen by a doctor, but this is not a bad thing. I am lying down with a nice, warm blanket and I can doze on and off as I please.

Tests. They need to take lots of tests: blood work, CAT scan, X-Rays. After a few hours the gastroenterologist on call sits down and holds my hand.

"You are a very sick lady, Mrs. Carley. We suspect you have cancer.'

What? What did he say? I have cancer?

I find out that two tumors have shown up on the CAT scan, both on my left side. I know this is spiritually significant, but cannot remember why. There may be more tumors lurking around inside me playing hide and seek with the technicians and their machines.

The blood work shows my intestines are too infected for a colonoscopy to be performed. I will have to be admitted upstairs to a room and the medical exams and further tests will proceed from there.

Holey Moley! I think, *I was at Saratoga Race Track five days ago having a wonderful time. How can this be happening to me!*

I realize these cancerous growths have not suddenly appeared today. They have been festering and growing for weeks and probably months. Something tipped the balance and now here I am facing the challenge of my life.

The admission process and in-take routine are blanks in my memory.

The first of many blanks to come.

My Spiritual Guides Have Something Big in Store For Me

I have just been figuratively whacked over the head by a 2X4.
What will happen to me now?
How will I care for my family?
Am I dying?

I am transported to the 5th floor of the hospital. My Reiki practitioner friends have gone home. They sat with me in the ER most of the day and their healing thoughts and prayers brought me the most caring, knowledgeable, medical staff who 'happened' to be on duty that day.

Later that night, after I am settled in, a guardian angel visited me disguised as the 'roommate from hell.'

She screamed, she cried, she begged, unsuccessfully, to be taken to the roof for a cigarette. She cried and screamed some more on her cell phone with her boyfriend claiming she was dying right this minute.

Hospital staff came and went. Nurses trying to get admitting information while calming her down. When asked for the name of her next of kin she screamed:

'Don't you dare call my father. I hate him.'

Her boyfriend finally comes in and gets into bed with her. I turn my TV way up to block out whatever is happening on the other side of the thin curtain.

In the morning while I am downstairs for yet another in a long series of tests, she is discharged. Just like that. Cured. Gone.

What a powerful lesson she was for me. I decided right then and there that I would not be my diagnosis. I would not let my illness rule my life. I would remain true to myself and experience what was happening to my body, but not change the essence of who I am.

I thanked and blessed this dear, neurotic stranger who zoomed into my world, carried on and on over essentially nothing, and zoomed out. I would not be like her.

Later that day another guardian angel took over the 'A' bed and gently guided me on my journey to physical and spiritual healing.

"Pssst, Patty, It's Time To Say the Rosary"

Each morning for the first week of my three week stay, my roommate woke me up at 7:28 a.m. with:

'Pssst, Patty, it's time to say the rosary with the TV.'

One of the nurses had brought me a specially blessed wooden rosary from Medjugorje so I was good to go.

We ate breakfast together on days I was not fasting for a test or blood work. Throughout the day we watched the same shows on our separate TVs. We watched 'Sister Act;' and laughed and laughed. We watched Oprah and cried and cried. At 4:00 p.m. we drank our bottles of Ensure.

"It's cocktail hour!" we declared.

The nurses said they loved coming into our room. It was a respite from the rest of the patients. We never complained and only rang the bell when we couldn't help one another ourselves.

As the days wore away and the strong IV antibiotics kicked in to kill the infection in my intestines, I was eating less and less. I had no strength to get out of bed and hadn't washed my hair in days. I wanted few to no visitors and after answering phone call after phone call from people who wanted information and the reassurances that I could not give them, I pulled the cord out of the wall and put the phone in the drawer. I wanted to think about my situation, to become immersed in the hospital routine, to make this place and this moment my only life. I barely thought about anyone outside these four walls.

My sister and husband were charged with telling family and friends I did not want visitors. People certainly wanted to see me and send me their love and good wishes, but I could not accept any of that at the time.

The staff assumed I was depressed and wanted to send in a social worker, a psychologist or a psychiatrist.

I said, 'No. I don't want to talk to anyone. Leave me alone.' Mercifully, they did.

I left cards unopened, plants unwatered, flowers unsmelled.

Nearly the only person I talked with was my angel roommate. She understood how I felt. She gently guided me through each day.

'Pssst, Patty. It's 3:28. Time to say the rosary on TV with Sister Angelica."

Ah....rosary beads and Ensure cocktails. It's Happy Hour at the Hospital.

Spirit Speaks To Me

I was sinking further down into myself. The strong antibiotics may have been killing the infection, but they were killing other things too. I developed thrush in my mouth and throat and now I could not swallow even the little bit I had been forcing myself to eat.

I lay in bed visualizing a clean colon. I sat up and practiced the Chi Gong movements to cure breast cancer while holding on to the window ledge. I said the rosary and asked God to please help me through this.

While waiting for my intestines to calm down enough to do the colonoscopy I had a mammogram, another CAT scan, a bone scan, an endoscopy and a breast biopsy, and, of course blood work, always blood work. I would cry when the technician from the blood lab came in the room, even when it was for my roommate.

For each test I had to fast and be sedated either mildly or more completely. I could feel my brain cells slipping away with each sedation.

One of the many tests I was given upon my arrival in the ER a week ago, showed a spot on my pancreas. The doctor delivering that bit of news was subdued and very concerned. He wanted to give me another test in a few days to get a better look. This would be a devastating diagnosis.

I had dreams and visions in which everything was crystal clear and in sharp focus. Was this due to my constant state of fasting? The strong antibiotics? Both? Neither?

I saw a beluga whale eating the cancer in my abdomen and saw the tumor in my left breast shrinking. I heard my personal Native American guide, Grandfather Spirit, speaking to me in my head.

'We will take the cancer in your pancreas away, but not the tumors in your breast and colon. You need these, little sister, to learn about medicine and healing. You must follow this path.'

'OK,' I whisper weakly, through my tears. 'I will do whatever you say. But will you at least hold my hand?'

'Yes, little sister, I will be right by your side.'

A few days later, after the endoscopy test to confirm the spot on my pancreas, my oncologist came in.

'The spot is gone. There must have been something wrong with the CAT scan machine in the ER.'

Thank you Grandfather Spirit. You kept your word.

Major Surgery and a Trip to the Afterlife

Perhaps a week has gone by and I can now have a colonoscopy. This is my first one, ever, and I am feeling so ill from everything else going on with me that I can barely choke down the prep solution. When the nurse finally leaves the room after watching me drink cup after cup of the awful tasting 'go-litely', I pour the rest on my plants. She is happy upon return to see I have finished it all. I have been a good girl, but will my plants survive?

Soon I am sitting on the commode next to my bed feeling nauseous and embarrassed because my roommate has several visitors who are talking and laughing on the other side of the thin curtain. I am groaning and crying and trying to not faint off the commode. It is a long night.

In the morning after I say the rosary, I wait and wait for them to take me downstairs for the colonoscopy. Of course, I can't have any breakfast or lunch and even though I am not hungry anyway I don't like it that it is forbidden. I am given a light anesthetic for the procedure and I tell the doctor he's cute as I drift away into a twilight state.

The colonoscopy shows that my situation is serious. The tumor is ready to push through my intestinal wall so.....I will be prepped the next morning for surgery in the evening. Surgery on a Friday night? This is sounding more and more dire.

The anesthesiologist visits me in the afternoon to discuss ways to put me under for the surgery. He strongly suggests I have an epidural IV put in my spine which will stay in for the pain medication afterwards. I agree that this sounds 'okay.' What do I know about these things anyway? I trust his judgment.

That little 'okay' sent me on a huge journey over the next few days.

I have scant memory of the time surrounding my abdominal surgery. I remember staring at the ceiling tiles in the hallways and elevator on my way down to the OR, then waking up in my room on the 5th floor on oxygen and in so much pain in spite of the morphine drip into my spinal column. I need to cough and am gagging and this hurts my incision so much I end up shouting.

Saturday is a drugged haze except for the intrusion of two nurses who walk into my room and say "Get up walking and wash yourself up."

"Huh?" I manage to whisper. "Who are you? Where am I?"

I am wearing leg compressors that whoosh and squeeze my lower legs in a constant, annoying rhythm and I cannot feel my feet at all. I am wearing a urine catheter and five wires and tubes attached to an IV pole, but up I go to shuffle to the door and back. What an exhausting trip!

The two nurses watch as I wash myself haphazardly with a wet cloth, breathe into a respirator tube, drink a few sips of water, choke and lay back down for a three hour nap.

By the wee hours of Sunday morning I am hallucinating sights and sounds. Bugs are crawling on the curtain, I hear sirens and imagine firemen breaking down my door with axes and coming to get me. I try to listen to my relaxation C Ds on my headphones but the voices are so slow and deep they scare me and I throw everything across the room.

I ring for the nurses every five minutes and, bless them, they come in to comfort me and give me anti-nausea shots and sips of ginger ale. At some point I feel myself in the funnel of a tornado and, like in the 'Wizard of Oz', people poke their heads and bodies through the swirling clouds to look at me. I see dead people, paralyzed people in wheelchairs, people I recognize and others I don't. I am swallowed up by the tornado and go down, down and around into darkness.

I like it there. It is calm and comforting. I want to stay there, but my beloved mentor Rita, who passed away three years before, sends me back up to the world. She tells me I have work to do on Earth and cannot be with her yet.

Oh, please, let me stay with you, This is all too painful for me.

"No. You have to go back," she says and gives me a not so gentle shove.

So, up and up I twirl and wake up in my hospital bed. I ring the bell yet again and ask the nurse to tell the person in the hall to stop screaming so I can get some sleep and she replies, "Honey, it's you who is screaming."

Now I know the morphine is doing bad things to my brain and I beg the nurses to call the surgeon and have this epidural thing taken out right now. It is 4:00 a.m. on Monday, but I must have been so insistent that the order comes through to have the drip stopped. Only the anesthesiologist can take the needle out when he comes in later in the day. I immediately start to feel calmer and the hallucinations slowly go away. When I become more aware of my surroundings I realize my angelic roommate is gone.

Why didn't she say goodbye? Was she ever here at all? Was she part of my hallucinations? How much time has passed?

I am alone in the room for a day or so until another woman is wheeled in after hip surgery. She is practically comatose so the room is bathed in silence. This is good. I am happy to be in silence. I say my rosary beads with the TV to myself. I feel my former roommate with me. Oh good, she was real after all.

Healing Comes My Way in Many Ways

During my three week hospital stay, unbeknownst to me, many people are praying for me, saying novenas, lighting candles, sending Reiki energy and folding origami peace cranes in my name.

A Shaman friend of mine, who is also a medical doctor, visits several times with her rattles, drum, feathers and a rain stick as tall as she is.

Each time she is with me my Oncologist 'happens' to stop by with good news to deliver: ' the colon surgery and resection was a success and you won't need a colostomy ,' 'the cancer has been contained,' 'there is no longer a spot on your pancreas,' 'you can go home soon to recuperate and get ready for the breast surgery in a month.'

He listens to the Shamanic ceremony and nods his head. I can hear the hospital staff stop outside my door and peer in.

'Something mysterious is going on in there!'

One day after my friend completes her ceremony, I lie back on the bed with my arms outstretched and think to myself:

I am a crossroads where Western and Eastern medicines meet. I have been given this experience to show others that both ways are necessary for healing. I am blessed.

As I begin to feel stronger my massage therapist comes in to give me a treatment, climbing over the bed and through the maze of tubes and wires. It feels divine.

Some of my Reiki practitioner friends stop by to give me energy.

All of these sessions help me to sit up for longer bits of time and eat tiny spoonfuls of beef broth, but my most pressing issue has become getting my hair washed.

It has been two weeks since I have washed my stringy, greasy, partially frosted, ½ gray hair. I can barely stand up alone and certainly cannot negotiate the tiny, triangular shower stall in my bathroom.

A nurse's aide comes by and asks if I need anything. I tell her about wanting to have my hair washed and itchy scalp scrubbed in the process. She tells me to wait, she has something to do first. About ½ hour later in she walks with a bucket, long hose, rectangular tray with a spout at one end and a plastic sheet. She found these in the hospital's basement and can now wash my hair while I lie in bed.

She closes the door and tells the rest of the staff to not disturb us for awhile, "I'm washing my Patty's hair."

Her kindness overwhelms me and my tears soon mingle with the shampoo running off my head into the bucket.

As I lie there with my eyes closed, enjoying the gentleness and peace, she quietly leaves the room. She has been an angel.

The doctors and nursing staff urge me at every meal to 'Eat, eat and get your strength back.'

I can barely choke down the warm vanilla pudding, yellow Jello, and flat ginger ale before crawling back into my bed. This bed that has become my safe haven, my cocoon. I don't ever want to leave it.

But, a few days later, I become brave enough to venture out of my room alone. I gather up the IV pole, catheter bag, leg compressor leads and head down to the nurses' station. The staff clap and cheer me on, so I stand a little straighter and walk one more step further to please my fans.

These are all steps on my path to healing. Each a different mode, but each an important part of the whole. I embrace them all.

Just One More Little Surgery

The next day when I ring the bell to find out where my breakfast tray is—I am actually hungry for it today—the nurse says I will be fasting that day in order to have surgery for an IV port to be inserted into the right side of my chest. This will be used for chemotherapy treatments, blood work, IV solutions, etc. The surgeon will also do a biopsy of my left breast to determine the extent of the cancer growing there.

Oh. I had almost forgotten about my left breast.

Later in the day, once again, I am given valium through an IV in my hand and I watch the ceiling tiles go by as I am wheeled into the OR.

An hour later, while in the Recovery area, I spy my surgeon writing notes at the desk."Hey you, Doc!" I shout much too loudly.

Everyone's head snaps up and I can hear a collective intake of breath. Who knows what a person coming out of anesthesia might say? I continue on boldly: "Every time you tell me I can eat real food, you do another procedure on me and I can't eat for two days."

He smiles and replies: "I keep dangling that carrot in front of you, don't I?" Everyone else smiles too. And I go back to sleep.

Going Home Too Soon

While waiting either to go into surgery or to recover from surgery, I have been watching a lot of television. The most interesting thing I noticed about television is the number of commercials and shows featuring food. Here I lie fasting every third day or so for some procedure or other and no matter what the TV show is about, there is food involved.

I can smell and taste the foods I see on the screen. Even foods I don't care for look delicious.

Another noteworthy observation is all the violence and crime on TV. If the show isn't some form of 'Law and Order,' it's the 5 o'clock, 6 o'clock, 7 o'clock, whatever o'clock news. Why is the majority of news bad, horrible, and bloody?

In the end I watched only 1960s reruns on TVLand, Sister Angelica and her rosary, and the Weather Channel.

By the time my hospital stay ended, Hurricane Katrina was barreling towards New Orleans and that was a horror/reality show of its own.

I found out that Wednesday that I would most likely be discharged by Friday.

What? So soon? I had surgery barely five days ago!

I called my sister in a panic. I wanted her to pick up Depends because I was still using a bedpan; lots of Jello and pudding because I wasn't eating real food yet; a hospital bed for the living room and on and on in my panic mode. I was frantic and crying.

How could I ever go home like this?

I obsessed about this all day and all that night.

However, the next morning, I awoke ravenous. I asked for a regular breakfast of pancakes, eggs, sausage and juice. I ate it all, Then I got up out of bed and walked, unaided, around the halls a few times, then washed my hair in the bathroom sink.

Friday, someone came in to take the IV lines out, the catheter out and the leg compressors off. I ate breakfast and walked around the halls again.

Saturday, my surgeon's partner came in for a routine check and I told him how great the food was here. He replied, "If you think this food is good, it is time for you to go home." He inspected the incision and yanked out the staples that I thought were staying in for another week. It's a good thing I didn't know he was going to do this. By the time my brain registered the pain, the staples were out. Smart man.

I called my husband and son to come get me and all my accumulated cards, flowers and extra juice boxes and, in a few hours, I was in the car heading home.

Home. What a strange thought. The car felt strange. My street looked strange. The flowers I had planted out front months before looked strange. The climb up the stairs felt strange and, with a few more shuffling steps, I was in my strange dining room. Suspended from the ceiling over the dining room table was a curtain of origami peace cranes my sister and Peace Pagoda friends had fashioned for me and hung from a birch tree branch.

I became overwhelmed by all that had happened to and for me. Finally, finally, I wept.

My Fuzzy Brain is Twirling, Earth's Energy is Swirling and A Butterfly Flutters By

Amazingly, I am taking no prescription pain killers at home, just Ambien to help me sleep at night. If I don't, the nightmares from the morphine overdose come back full force.

I have trouble focusing on anything: conversations, television, books, crossword puzzles. Once people realize I am home they want to come over, call, send cards and flowers. It is all wonderful and comforting to be so loved, but overwhelming at the same time. How can I carry on a normal conversation without crying? How can I act like everything is okay when I don't know if it is or ever will be?

Every morning I make myself get out of bed, get showered—which is a slow, unsteady process— put on decent clothes and make-up. It becomes my link back to reality, the make-up and clean hair.

I eat very small portions of comfort foods and Ensure in the afternoons. I reminisce about 'cocktail hour' at the hospital with my angelic roommate.

Hurricane Katrina is bearing down on New Orleans. All that swirling energy exploding through the Gulf of Mexico. I am glued to CNN and coming unglued emotionally watching this tragedy unfold. My fuzzy brain cannot take it all in as I get sucked into the vortex of the horror and grief before me.

This twirling hurricane is similar to the vortex I was being sucked into during my morphine overdose a week ago. Was my experience in the hospital a foreshadowing of Katrina? Was my energy center picking up on the swirling energy still a few days out in my future? I know these experiences are connected, just not how. It hurts my head to think about it.

I switch the TV off.

A monarch butterfly keeps fluttering around the second floor living room window when I am sitting there and around the flowers when I am sitting on my front porch. Butterflies signify transformation, going through the stages of pupa, larva, cocoon, then beautiful butterfly.

Is this what I just experienced in the hospital?

Does this butterfly signify my own transformation?

My own rebirth?

It hurts my head to think about this.

I switch my brain off.

More Tests, More Surgery. More Transformations

The end of September, 2005 is fast approaching and my doctors feel I am ready for the breast surgery they have put off until my colon surgery and recovery were complete. How I can be completely healed from major surgery in three weeks is mysterious. I don't feel completely healed, but I trust they know what they are doing.

I have to be at the hospital at 7:30 a.m. for some procedure in advance of the scheduled lumpectomy. I wait two hours for this procedure to take place and wish it had never happened at all.

With no anesthesia, no valium and no pain killer on the site, a young man—a technician? a doctor?— poked four needles full of blue, radioactive dye into my tender breast tissue to help the surgeon see the lump, lymph nodes and any escapee cancer cells.

'This will only hurt a little. Believe me, a needle with Novacain would hurt more.'

Are you kidding me? This is the worst pain I have had to withstand so far.

My body has forgotten the pain after the abdominal surgery. My clever brain has removed memories of that intense pain.

During the procedure I tried to go through the Tai Chi movements in my head. Couldn't.

I tried to get to my 'happy place' in my head. Couldn't.

Finally, I asked my spirit guide to come hold my hand and he did. With tears streaming off the right side of my face and making a puddle on the floor at the doctor's feet, I prayed my way through the procedure and was able to check off my list another unasked for invasion of my body.

I was sent home for 1 ½ hours and then went back to Nuclear Medicine (now there's an ominous sounding name) to have pictures taken of my breast which was a piece of cake procedure. Everything is relative to the procedure before.

From Nuclear Medicine I walk down to the out-patient OR.

Out-patient? How can surgery with the words 'removal of damaged body parts' in it be considered out-patient?

I am led into the OR and given a 'johnny coat' to put on for the surgery. I am naked underneath except for socks and underpants which I joke about with the nurses. They hook me up to an IV through my chest port. Thank goodness for that—no more vein poking.

I say hi to the surgeon and tell him we have to stop meeting like this. I can see his eyes smiling above his mask in agreement.

I hoist myself onto the operating table in the glare of the overhead lights and ask if they are going to be putting me to sleep for this procedure. The anesthesiologist laughs and tells me to count to ten. I get to number 1 ½ and wake up in the recovery room.

Why are these places always so brightly lit? It hurts my eyes.

The nurse gives me a codeine pill I don't want and when she offers me another I refuse. Pain is relative to the previously experienced pain and this is not as bad as the blue-dye needles.

I am hungry, is what I am. Ravenous. They bring me saltine crackers and ginger ale.

"Hey, this isn't food," I shout.

My husband is coming to pick me up at 5 p.m.

While waiting, I tell the nurses about all the Reiki energy and prayers sent my way and they agree it helps enormously with the healing process. I am glad to hear the healing practices are filtering into the medical profession. At least the nurses are noticing.

On the way out the door one nurse yells to me to not be alarmed if my urine is blue for 24 hours. Thank goodness she remembered to tell me, I peed bright blue for hours and would have been scared.

I had been in the OR and recovery area for only four hours and am leaving with ½ a breast missing, the lumpectomy turning into a partial mastectomy.

They tell me to call them if I notice anything different or feel strange. Of course I feel strange. Part of my body is missing. This has been the last of six surgical procedures of one kind or another in as many weeks and I should call if I feel different or strange?

Everything feels different and strange!

My life is different and strange.

Who am I now?

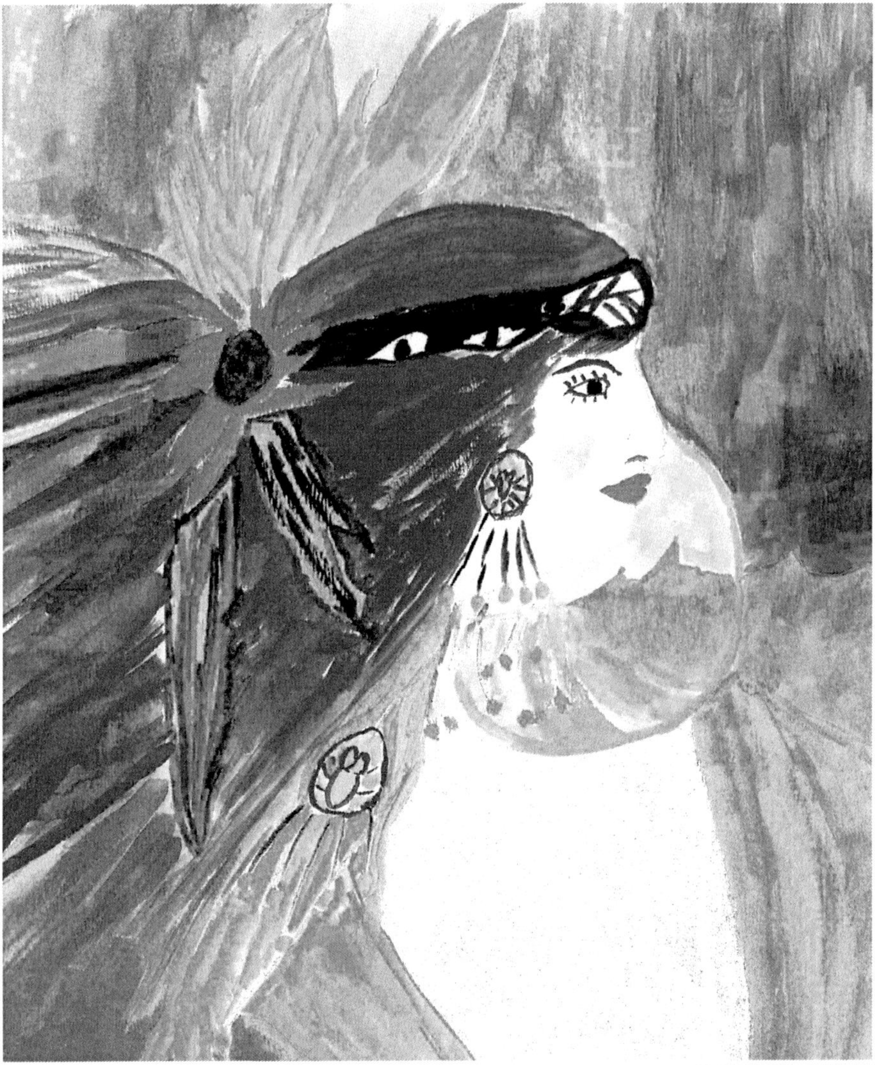

© PATRICIA CARLEY

Female Warrior

From the dim past,
in the far reaches of our minds,
we recall stories of a tribe of women.
Warriors. Protectors.
Who cut off a breast, right or left,
so they could pull the bowstring
unfettered by flesh.
Mastectomies for power and strength,
to protect what was theirs from harm.
Did I hear them reach out to me?
Call to me? Sing to me?
'Remember our lives.
Remember our sacrifices
in order to secure the life you live today.
Tell our story. Teach our ways.
Become a Warrior without your breast.
Able to stand tall, not mutilated and small
But forever whole and strong.'

Physical Therapy for Physical Strength, Spiritual Therapy for Spiritual Strength

In retrospect, the easier part is over. Each surgery and recovery period is relative to the previous one. The body heals at its own pace and one recovers, or not, as time goes by.

The grueling part is about to begin. The therapies and post-cancer treatments and drugs await me. Good thing I don't know what to expect.

My Oncologist and Radiologist confer and decide I am strong enough to do radiation and chemo therapies simultaneously so they don't stretch into a year-long process.

"OK," I say. They are the experts after all and I will follow their advice.

Besides my fuzzy brain believes I am up for this challenge.

Bring it on. I think.

I have already begun physical therapy sessions to strengthen the muscles around my left breast. I cannot reach with that arm yet, so closing the car door is a challenge and I have to carry everything in my right hand. The therapist remarks how I am her only patient who does the therapy at home between sessions.

I want to be strong and healthy for the upcoming post-cancer treatments.

Physical therapy for physical strength.

I need to go into this with a good attitude, too.

I read my favorite spiritual authors: Wayne Dyer, Rumi, Louise Hay, Richard Bachman, Dan Milliman and Neale Donald Walsch. Their every word holds meaning for me.

I talk on the phone with my spiritual mentors and friends and they each enlighten me in interesting ways.

One friend gave me a new twist on the morphine overdose I experienced after the colon surgery. She explained how drugs were used by native people to help them cross into the spirit realm, thus my morphine 'overdose' and subsequent spiral into the swirling vortex of the spirit world. I had figuratively and probably literally been lost to this reality for three days during my hallucinations. I was obtaining information from my spirit guides and needed to withdraw from the physical world and stay focused on what my soul was receiving on another plane.

Since my spirit guides could not get me to go on a vision quest in the traditional way, they sent me on one any way they could.

Wow! Thank you, my friend, for this valuable insight.

This completely changed how I looked at this experience. I was no longer angry with the anesthesiologist for overdosing me. He was the instrument through which I was sent on a journey necessary to my personal growth. I had always been curious about vision quests. I wonder what I learned during mine.

As the end of October approaches I make an appointment to get my left breast 'mapped' for radiation treatments. This map will be a guideline for the technicians to follow so the beam from the radiation machine will hit the right spots.

That day I have a telephone session with my spiritual mentor. We visualize the radiation treatments as a day at the beach in the Bahamas. A beach of white sand and turquoise water with gentle waves lulling me to sleep. The rays from the machine will be the rays of the sun, infusing me with the strength and energy to withstand the upcoming months of intense treatments.

Spiritual therapy for spiritual strength.

Trick or Treat

The chemo-therapy treatments begin on October 31st. There are layers of meaning in this for me. I remember from my Catholic upbringing that it is All Souls' Day. It is a day to dress up and pretend to be someone else. It is a day to wear a mask and ask for treats. It is a day to play tricks on others if they don't give us what we ask for.

What will I be asked to do today at the doctor's office? Will the ensuing treatments turn me into someone else once again? Will my real self be unmasked?

The Radiologist wanted to start me on treatments today also, but agreed to start November 1st, All Saints' Day. This seems to be a good plan since I can use help from *all* the Saints.

I arrive at my Oncologist's office at 9 a.m. Today and every treatment day I make it a priority to be well-dressed with make-up and a smile on my face. I don't know what will happen to me today, but at least I will be wearing a mask with a happy face.

Before I am hooked up to the chemo-therapy IVs the nurse recites all the dos and don'ts associated with treatments sessions. It is a long list of foods to eat or avoid, advice to stay away from anyone with a cold, avoiding restaurants and no eating at salad bars at all, keeping drinks room temperature, using plastic utensils because the metallic components in the chemo will emphasize the cold and leave a bad taste in my mouth, on and on and on.

My fuzzy brain cannot retain all this information, so instead I totally focus on the fact that I will most likely lose my hair. This is all I can think about, obsess about, cry about. It is the final outrage against my body. It will mark me as 'someone in treatment for cancer.' I am devastated.

I say I understand everything that was said to me, but I don't.

The nurse then leaves the room to get my infusion supplies and the woman sitting next to me already hooked up to an IV suddenly turns scarlet, clutches her throat and whispers, 'I can't breathe.' I call for help. No one comes. I call again, then realize I am not hooked up to anything and can run for help, which I do. The medical staff rush in and get her stabilized, then start up my chemo treatments. What a way to begin my day. I am nervous about what just happened to someone else. Can this happen to me, too?

I am in the treatment room for five hours, not three like I was told, and have not eaten all day. I am exhausted, headachy, scared and worried about the fanny pack I have to wear for three more days that attaches a chemo drip into my port through a machine that whooshes and clicks night and day. How will I sleep without rolling over onto the pack and shutting it off?

I finally get home, try to eat some mashed potatoes and take ½ an Ambien to make sure I sleep, but not too soundly, so I don't roll over onto the fanny pack.

The next morning I begin radiation treatments at the hospital.

I have to lie absolutely still but I can visualize that white beach in the Bahamas and float away while the machine whirs and clicks over me and the fanny pack I wear whooshes and clicks under me. I am lying naked to the waist while a male technician scans my breast and underarm. I think about how horrified my mother would be if she had to do this. I say to myself that I am having these treatments for all the women who cannot. They are being healed through me.

Just as I visualize the sun during the radiation treatments, I visualize the chemo drugs as the elixir of life. I do not think of them as poison, as I have been told they are. I do not see the chemo drugs killing bad cells in my body. Rather, I see this life-giving serum filling me with golden light and transforming errant, malfunctioning cells into perfect, life-giving cells. I think about embracing this healing moment.

This keeps me uplifted, serene and sane.

So, are these cancer therapies a Trick or a Treat? It depends upon the day and how strong I feel emotionally at any given time.

Will 2006 be a Happy New Year?

My radiation treatments are completed on December 28th. I have become friends with the staff and feel conflicted about leaving this cocoon of healing energy, just as I felt conflicted about leaving the hospital in August. Each transition is a little bit scary. Heading off into the unknown each time.

My Oncologist gave me three weeks off from chemo-therapy treatments so I can rest up for a few days. My husband had knee surgery before Christmas and we both needed a break from medical procedures.

Now we could welcome in 2006 or worry about what 2006 might bring.

My 5th chemo treatment is on January 3rd. I get hooked up to the IV and settle back in the lounge chair. I nod hello to the lady and her husband sitting across from me and start my daily meditation that puts me in a good frame of mind. Around 20 minutes into the treatment, I feel hot and look at my hands which are bright red. I am hyper-ventilating, my blood is pounding in my ears and I am suddenly nauseous. I look at the man sitting near me and find all I can do is whisper, 'Help. Please help me.'

The doctor who has been filling in for my vacationing Oncologist comes rushing in with the nurse and the last thing I remember after they pull out the IV line, shoot in Benadryl and wrap a blood pressure cuff on me is her saying 'At least she's still breathing.'

I pass out.

When I awake, which turns out to be three hours later, I am disoriented, alone and ravenous.

"Hey, is anyone here?" I shout out.

The nurse runs in to see if I am OK and I ask her to find me some food and the T.V. clicker so I can watch "Dallas."

I'm in luck, the drug reps were in earlier and left a platter from Panera. However, Dallas has been off the air for ten years.

"Ten years? Really?"

I eat a sandwich and fall back to sleep for another three hours. Now it is evening, all the patients and most of the staff have left and I'm ready to go home. The problem is they won't let me drive because of all the Benadryl in my system, my husband can't drive yet and my fuzzed brain cannot think of one person to pick me up.

I start to cry. "I have no friends. There is no one to come get me."

I cannot think of my neighbors' names, my in-laws names, my own sister's name. Any number of people would come get me, but I can think of no one.

About an hour later, my Oncologist's wife, even though on vacation, comes to drive me home. I cry and thank her profusely all the way to my house. She assures me she is happy to do this.

In the midst of all this turmoil and trauma, I get a phone call that my son John had a drop seizure and is in the Emergency Room. They assure me he is being well taken care of.

I am so involved with my own situation, I tell them to just call me when he gets back to his residence. I cannot begin to deal with this.

For good or for ill, we are roaring into 2006. One of my resolutions is to learn to 'embrace the moment' I am experiencing, but can I do this?

Animals as Therapists, Writing as Therapy

My chocolate Lab, Ruffy, is my constant companion. She sniffs my left armpit and nuzzles my abdomen. She senses that something is different with me. I think she can smell the chemo drugs and feel the burned areas of my breast and underarm. We take leisurely walks together in the mornings and evenings and it is nice to not have to talk. I don't have to explain myself to her.

In February I take my son Dan to a doctor's appointment. The doctor's dog, a black Spaniel named Rochester, is on duty that day. As we wait in the examining room, Rochester noses his way in the door, comes right up to me and puts his paws on my lap. His eyes are level with mine and he looks deeply into them for several moments, no blinking.

I hear a voice in my head. "You are healed."

Rochester gets down and leaves the room.

As it turns out, Dan doesn't need any medical attention so I know this visit has been for me and Rochester. Spirit has spoken through him.

When I visit my Shaman friend, her dogs come into her healing room. One lies under the table and the other puts his paws on areas of my body that need attention. She follows his lead with placing her crystals and feathers around my body.

In the midst of my new life shaped by office visits, treatments and follow-ups, I manage to continue writing and mailing a monthly newsletter that my mentor, Rita, started over 20 years ago. I hear from many people how my current poems and writings have helped them or someone they know deal with difficulties in their lives. I am so grateful that I can do this. It helps me to help others. It is healing for me to share my experiences with cancer and show how these experiences can be handled with humor and good grace.

I don't feel called to do anything "big" such as climbing a mountain, running a marathon or sky diving. I seem to be finding smaller, more individualized ways to serve humankind. I feel guided to help the person right in front of me, which spirit assures me will ripple out to touch many, many more.

Here is my list of reasons why my experience with cancer was a gift:

10. I learned to let go of my fears and embrace the moment
9. Prayers are answered
8. I met and received care from wonderful medical professionals
7. I am learning to say 'no' to things I cannot or will no longer do.
6. I am learning to be a 'human being' instead of a 'human doing'
5. I learned many things about my body—mostly how to honor it through the surgeries and treatments and not be attached to the outcome
4. I came to realize how much love from family and friends there is for me. WOW!
3. I can help others navigate the cancer network
2. I learned to embrace cancer, not battle it
1. I don't have to have my facial hair waxed as often

Chemo Ends and I Have a Revelation

I resume chemo treatments after a week of rest to help my battered body refresh and renew. The offending drug is withdrawn from the 'cocktail' I have been on and stay with the one that requires the wearing of the fanny pack for three days. I can now sleep through the whoosh—click for a few hours at a time.

One day my doctor's son stops by the infusion room as I am having a treatment. He is becoming a doctor himself and is spending the day with his dad. When they stop to talk to me I am introduced in terms of my symptoms, surgical procedures and chemical treatments. This is so upsetting to me I just have to say something.

"Excuse me. I know you are doctors and this is how you discuss your patients with one another, but I want you to know I am NOT my diagnosis. I am NOT my symptoms. I am NOT my treatments. I am a person experiencing cancer, not the cancer itself. It is just one small part of who I am. Hi. My name is Pat Carley." And I extend my hand.

They immediately apologize and thank me for saying this. They sometimes get caught up in the medical, and diagnostic details.

I thank Spirit for giving me this opportunity to remind medical practitioners that we patients are people first and our diagnoses a distant second.

I have no more adverse reactions to the chemo drugs and on April 18, 2006 I have my last treatment. I buy myself a new, red car with a 'moon roof.'

I am able to resume Tai Chi classes a few weeks later and I receive an amazing insight. My teacher is talking about the 'Dantien,' the place in the lower abdomen where our energy flows or is stopped up. I realize it is right where my surgery scar is! I had been surgically opened up so the stagnant energy trapped in there could be released. New energy can now flow through my re-sectioned bowel area, my bone marrow can be cleansed with this new energy and I can start to 're-member' who I am.

This is Only a Test . . .

'This is a test. This is only a test of the emergency broadcast system. Do not adjust your set.' These words lept into my mind as I now have to face post-cancer tests.

I need a PET/CAT scan to see if all the cancer has been radiated, burned and chemoed out of me these past six months.

Sounds like a friendly enough test, 'pet cat.'

I fast from midnight the night prior to the test. Now, there's a strange word. Fast. Without food the time goes by very slowly indeed.

Upon arrival at the medical lab I wait and wait in the well-named Waiting Room. Finally a white-coated woman takes me to a cubicle for a short consultation. She has to keep the door open to this room because she admits to being claustrophobic. In 30 minutes I will appreciate the humor in this.

After waiting some more, wearing one of those goofy hospital gowns that I still cannot get my arms into on the first try, I am taken to another small room where I have to drink a pint of liquid which is white, thick and difficult to swallow. I wait until the technician leaves and pour ½ of it down the sink as there are no plants in the room. When he returns I smile and announce, 'All gone.' I have been a good girl once again.

He needs to start an I.V. drip. No problem. I have a port in my chest for just such an occasion. However, no one on duty is authorized to access it.

Are they kidding me? This is exactly why I have the port!

He has to repeatedly poke my right arm to find a suitable vein. They are hard and small from all the chemo drugs and I am now ready to throw-up and/or leave. Finally, after I am made to feel this has all been somehow my fault , a vein is found and I can go to the next step. How much worse can it get? Just you wait!

I lie down on a very narrow board and am strapped down chest to feet.

"Don't move a muscle or we will have to start over." I am instructed.

The CAT machine whizzes over me and takes whatever pictures it needs and I think, *This will be a piece of cake, which is good since I have to pee really badly after drinking all those fluids.*

"Hah!" I hear inside my head.

The technician goes into another room and turns on a Frank Sinatra CD much too loudly and I slowly, ever so slowly begin to be pulled into a very narrow, completely enclosed tube.

I realize immediately that I cannot rationally handle this. I have to get my spirit self out of this tube or I will go mad. Where can I go? What can I think about? How can I stop obsessing about having to pee?

It occurs to me I can visualize Tai Chi in my head. I go over all three sections very slowly. Finished with that. Fifteen minutes down. *Now what?* I open my eyes a slit to see how far in the tube I am and cannot see light at either end.

Oh, Mother of God, help me. I cannot do this alone.

I have no feeling in my hands, feet or really any part of my bound body now except my bladder. Then She comes to me. Mary, the Blessed Mother. She recites the rosary with me as, with miniscule movements, I count the Hail Marys on my fingers. The rosary is finished now, too. Another fifteen minutes gone.

I know I am going to scream right now! And suddenly I hear a disembodied voice —maybe it's Frank Sinatra?—say: 'You're done.'

And I whiz out of the tube feet first.

I have been bound into this machine so tightly I can barely walk and can't talk. I make it to the bathroom without a moment to spare. I never should have driven myself here. I am hungry, nauseous and can feel a migraine cranking up.

I drive through Dunkin Donuts to get anything with sugar on it and laugh to myself about the employee back there who had claustrophobia in the dressing room, for Pete's sake!

I congratulate myself for finding a way to stay inside the PET machine without screaming. I was able to embrace the moment through prayer and visualizations. However, I am never doing this test again without serious medication.

As I recover from cancer surgeries, treatments and post-cancer tests I am learning more about how to live my life.

Here follows another Top Ten list:

10. Chocolate is a food group with magical healing powers.

9. I will wear a skirt that twirls at least once a week.

8. I ask God each day to make me a blessing to someone.

7. I make plans no more than 1 day in advance, if that.

6. Saying kind words and gossiping less is a better way to communicate.

5. I am no longer waiting in line to eat a meal no matter how renowned the restaurant.

4. I can best share my experiences by just being them.

3. Life is perfect just the way it is. Stop trying to control everything!

2. I am listening to my body and spirit. They are smarter than my brain.

1. If the electricity goes out, eat the ice cream first and feed the melting meatballs to the dog.

New Parts For a New Me

As it turned out, I didn't need a wig. All that obsessing and crying for nothing. What I did need was a haircut and my gray hair colored. During chemo-therapy I was advised to not get a perm nor my hair frosted. Too many chemicals were in my system already so who knew what color my hair might turn?

The day of my last infusion I called my hair stylist for an appointment and became a short-haired blonde, once more. I saved $15 for waxing since my eyebrows and upper lip hair had not grown back yet.

Now that the swelling in my left breast was down I saw I was in need of some padding and new bras. The lingerie store I went to specialized in just these items. The owner measured me, assessed my naked upper body, had me turn this way and that and then popped a fake breast into the pocket of a bra and pulled a t-shirt over my head. When I turned around to see myself in the mirror, I cried. The bra felt so good. Both sides of my chest were in alignment. I looked good in a tight t-shirt. I felt back in balance. The owner and I hugged and cried some more.

I was also back to wearing pants with a waistband and zipper instead of stretchy elastic. The next body parts to give me trouble were my teeth. Over a two-year period I had one extraction, two crowns, two root canals and several fillings redone. Radiation and chemo along with hormone drugs created their own hurricane in my mouth.

In July, 2007 I had the IV port removed from my chest. This signified to me that I was finished with treatments and would not be going back.

The radiation burns were fading. The scars were healing. Less and less I needed to always know where the nearest bathroom was located. I could drink cold water right out of the tap. (Not too cold, though).

I embraced it all and thanked God and my Spirit guides I was alive.

Living Beyond Cancer

It has been six years since my diagnosis, surgeries, treatments and subsequent cure. It has taken me this long to be able to look at that first year and try to make some sense of it all.

My fellow-patients and I joked about 'chemo-brain,' but the truth is I have lost brain cells to anesthesia and cancer treatments and they are not coming back. I have had to find new ways to retain information and memories. I have to check and re-check my spelling and grammar when writing anything.

I have to admit that some things from my former life are just gone. However, this loss has also opened up new space for new ideas and new activities to come in.

I learned how to paint with watercolors.

This is the third book I have written and published in the past three years.

I study and practice Reiki, yoga and Tai Chi.

I even jog around the block once in awhile.

I have follow-up medical examinations, blood work, mammograms and colonoscopies.

Over the past few years, I have been discharged from the care of some of my doctors. I am healthy now and have mostly routine office visits with the remaining ones.

God spared me for a reason I have yet to fully realize. I have glimpses of why I am still alive. I know I need to share what I went through and discovered about medical care, 'alternative' care and how the blending of many healing practices brought me to this day.

I sit outside on a warm summer's night. I gaze up at the sky, squinting to find the Beehive cluster in the constellation Cancer. I ponder the immensity of the Universe and my place in it.

I think about all that has been taken away from me and all that I have been given and I am grateful for both.

I embrace the moment with joy.

About the Author

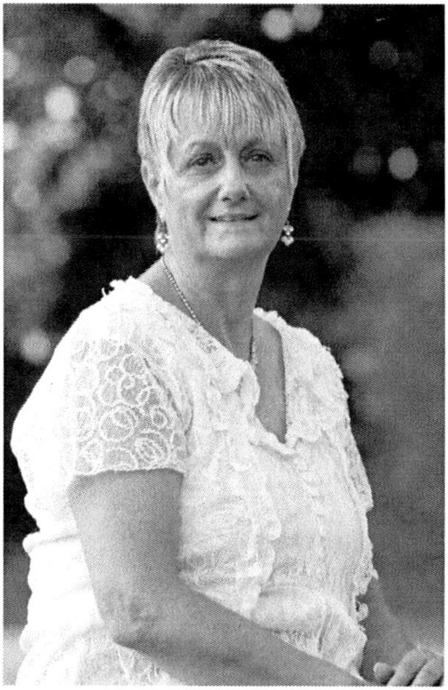

Patricia Carley began writing stories and poetry at an early age. When she was nine one of her poems was published in a local school newsletter and thus began her passion for seeing her thoughts in print.

As a student at SUNY Binghamton, where she received a BA in English Literature, and throughout the next 40 years Patricia continued to write and publish poetry and serve as editor of several newsletters.

In 2008 she was inspired to write a historical novel, *My Grandmother's Necklace,* about her Hungarian grandmother's journey to America in 1912. The next year she published the book, *Heart to Heart,* chronicling the life of her developmentally challenged son John and his ability to touch people's hearts through his art work.

Patricia has helped raise funds for local charitable organizations through the sale of her books. She has spoken at book clubs, local libraries and book stores, and facilitated creative writing workshops at area literacy programs.

Dreamweaver, the sequel to *My Grandmother's Necklace,* will be available in 2012.